Ten Hypnoses. Volume 1: Psychooncology

Ingo Michael Simon

TEN HYPNOSES

Hypnotherapy manual instructions and session scripts

Volume 1
Psychooncology

Imprint

Copyright © 2021 Ingo Michael Simon

Translation: PH.D. Hanne E. Jahn, Netherlands
published by IS Media eG, Germany
Website: www.ingosimon.com

ISBN: 9798749059700
Independently published

All rights reserved; no part of this publication may be reproduced or transmitted by any means, electronic, mechanical, photocopying or otherwise, without the prior permission of the publisher.

IMPORTANT NOTE

Ingo Michael Simon studied psychology plus educated pedagogy and is a hypnotherapist with practical work in southwest Germany and Switzerland. With the help of hypnosis-assisted psychotherapy, he primarily treats people with persistent psychological ailments, anxiety disorders, pathological compulsions and psychosomatic diseases form the focus of his practice. His therapeutic offers mainly include classic and modern hypnosis applications, regression and reincarnation therapy as well as therapy on the magic meadow and the dreamland therapy he developed himself. That is why he developed therapy sequences that he wrote down in over 200 books on a topic-related basis.

The contents of this book are based on the authors' practical experience with hypnosis and psychotherapy in a state of trance. Although the authors have taken the greatest possible care, errors or misunderstandings in the presentation cannot be completely ruled out. Therapeutic work with people and the use of hypnosis are the sole responsibility of the hypnotist. It cannot be ruled out that parts of this book may be misunderstood or that the use of a procedure presented may cause an undesirable reaction in the client. The authors also do not share the responsibility when working with a client with reference to the explanations in this book.

This series of books makes every day work with patients easier for every therapist. You no longer need to write your own texts and this save a lot of time that can be used for patients in your practice. In the German-speaking countries these books are bestsellers, which now lead to the knowledge and experience being brought onto the international market. PH. D. Hanne E. Jahn now translates these books step by step into several languages. She runs her practice for psychotherapeutic hypnosis in several languages in the Netherlands, with international patients.

COPYRIGHT AND USE

With this book/program you get texts written by me, Ingo Michael Simon (Dipl.-Päd. univ. trained psychologist and practitioners for psychotherapy), were written personally and translated by Hanne E. Jahn.

I point to it: point out that even with texts that are passed on as WORD documents or PDFs, the Copyright applies in the same way as it does to printed books. What does that mean exactly? The following uses of the texts are expressly permitted by me personally: - Use in work with your own clients - Electronic storage, for example copying in WORD for individual processing, if the texts are to be adapted for your own work with clients - Sound recording of the texts during the therapy session or outside of it when the recording is given to a client (to support the therapy)- Sound recording to listen to the texts yourself. However, the following uses are not permitted:

- Publication of the texts under your own name
- Selling the texts, not even giving them away for free
- Reproduction of sound recordings for commercial use (publication and Sale); A sound recording may only be sent to a client as part of a treatment to be passed on!
- Publishing or making available to the public an audio recording of the texts on the internet (youtube, homepage etc.)
- Lending or copying of the texts for passing on to others

Any use that is not expressly approved beyond the lawful use requires the consent of the authors, in this case our personal written consent Approval. I ask all customers to observe and respect the copyright. Thank you very much for your understanding and your support! Your Ingo Michael Simon!

TABLE OF CONTENTS

The modular system 9
The main part texts 10
Introduction 1: 13
Introduction 2: 15
Introduction 3: 16
Deepening of trance 1: 17
Deepening of trance 2: 18
Deepening of trance 3: 19
Promotion of willingness to change (compliance) 1: For those affected 20
Promotion of willingness to change (compliance) 2: For those affected 21
Promotion of willingness to change (compliance) 3: For relatives 22
Main Part 1: Persevering in Chemotherapy 23
Main part 2: Accompany chemotherapy 27
Main part 3: activate self-healing power 31
Main part 4: activate self-healing power 35
Main Part 5: Soap Bubbles against Cancer 39
Main part 6: Addressing the body 43
Main part 7: activate self-healing power 47
Main Part 8: Mindfulness and Healing 51
Main Part 9: The Flow of Life 55
Main Part 10: Making Peace 59
Transition to rejection 1: 63
Transition to rejection 2: 64
Transition to diversion 3: 65
Rejection 1: 66
Rejection 2: 67
Rejection 3: 68
Book series coming soon: 69

Forwarding, publication & copying in any form is prohibited and subject to compensation.

Copying, publishing and passing on to third parties is prohibited and only permitted with the written consent of the author Ingo Simon. Please carefully observe the information on copyright and use.

The modular system

On the one hand, I wrote this book to give ideas, examples within reach and to show how hypnosis can actually look like in everyday practice. On the other hand it is but also designed as a reading or, more precisely, reading book. Because nothing at all speaks against reading a hypnosis text. It doesn't make him worse.

The structure and process of hypnosis is described differently by different authors and trainers, although most of them follow the same basic idea. I prefer not only simple processes, but also comprehensible structures and therefore distinguish seven steps of a hypnosis session in this series of books. There are texts templates for each step that follow can be combined with each other as desired. I chose this structure despite being finished templates also leave room for individuality. Over time, or for advanced hyperchess, it becomes easier to use their own texts and formulations and only to take the main part of the respective session from this book. I distinguish the following steps on Hypnosis:

1. Introduction (induction)
2. Deepening the trance
3. Promotion of willingness to change (compliance)
4. Main part (therapy part, application part)
5. Consolidation (post-hypnotic assignment)
6. Transition to diversion
7. Elimination of the trance

The points in the texts ... ... interrupt ... ... the ... ... reading flow and force you to take break or to reading slowly, which is usually much more difficult than hands-free speaking. Build the texts in. Read them in and read them out or change parts of them and adapt them for your clients. Generally valid text templates that have the same effect on all clients and all problem constellations cannot be created. I don't understand my books that way either. I understand you especially as collections of examples, which in many cases, are confirmed by numerous communications from me Readers, are already suitable or can be made suitable by adding a few individual and personalized additions. But I also see them as templates that serve as the basis of own texts and suggestions can serve. Decide for yourself.

The main part texts

In the texts for the main parts, I made sure to offer different forms of hypnosis. In my own work, the therapy sessions often contain elements from different areas that I combine with one another, for example I incorporate ide motoric communication into imaginary journeys. In the series *Ten Hypnoses* I use the following and many other variants of hypnosis: Classic suggestions, Anchor technology, Creative association, Ide motoric skills, Somatic-emotional therapy, Fantasy trip, Suggestion of increase, Affirmation hypnosis, I-suggestion, Guided self-instruction, Timeline hypnosis, Regression hypnosis, Suggestion of increase, Sensory focus, Self-hypnosis triggers, Insistent suggestion, Hidden instruction, Intentional suggestion, Mirror suggestion (first person), Suggestion stairs, Dog walking method, Causal suggestion, Narrative hypnosis, Symbol imagination, Dissociative trance, Suggestive triple jump, Reframing, Dreamland therapy

In this book you will find texts on the following variants of hypnosis:

- Classic suggestion
- Anchor technology
- Creative association
- Ide motor work
- Somatic-emotional visualization
- Dreamland therapy

The two text templates for *classic suggestion* work with constructive formulations, the work on a linguistic-logical basis and formulated according to describable suggestion rules become. It depends on formulations that promote a constructive attitude and confirm the inner focus on the therapeutic goal. If you want to take a closer look at the formulation rules for suggestions, you will find detailed information with many examples in my book *Formulating Suggestions Correctly*.

Anchoring techniques work with conditioned, i.e. trained or learned signals that are supposed to trigger a certain feeling, thought or perception. The anchor can be, for example, a body movement, a symbol or talisman that is looked at or a scent that is absorbed through the nose.

Creative associations are pictorial representations of scenes that symbolize the problem being dealt with and are understood and changed as a substitute for it. These hypnoses are less about sophisticated formulations than about the plasticity of the visualizations.

With the, *ide motor communication*, receive feedback from the client's body, which externally depicts internal processes via visible signals such as finger movements or arm levitations, reddening of the skin or catalepsies (immobility). It is important not to query any active signals from the client, but to use unconsciously controlled and unconsciously given signals.

Somatic-emotional hypnoses work with the connection between emotion and body awareness and guide changes controlling the focus on and mindfulness for one's own body. For quick orientation, a subtitle is of course printed with each main part of the text, which shows which variant it is in each case.

Go on imaginary journeys finally a long way over several stations of an imagined world in order to get into this to deal with problems in the fantasy world and to find solutions. For this variant for hypnosis, I offer texts from the dreamland therapy I developed, which are the actual stories are not structured in terms of content, as is the case with many fantasy trips or trance stories is common. The Land of Dreams is more like a film set with open scenes that are intuitively filled by the client's memory and visualized emotions.

At this point I would like to point out that books cannot replace therapies. To of course, psychotherapy or other therapeutic treatment takes more than that, a careful diagnosis is the necessary basis for decision-making for the use of the funds, also for whether hypnosis or one of my texts may be used. But also in this one case include preliminary talks, follow-up talks during the session and of course a therapeutic one concept of the sequence of sessions and the content-related procedure for a therapy. I can and cannot afford a collection of texts. Deep internal conflicts and pathological conditions must always be viewed in their entirety and complexity. Educates in my practical work Carl Rogers' talk therapy forms the basis of the client's inner conflict with himself and his subjects. Supplement guided fantasy trips or other hypnosis treatments this work and help the client to recognize and work on what is difficult to access or completely blocked to his waking consciousness. So simple the texts of the book partly this may sound like it is not embedded in structured and professionally conducted psychotherapy necessary to use more complex or delicately formulated and intensely suggestive hypnosis. In simplicity is much more often the possibility of actual change. At least that corresponds to my experience as a naturopath for psychotherapy, with daily work.

Introduction 1:

... ... Find the most comfortable position ... ... so comfortable that it seems like it is hardly possible anymore more comfortable ... ... as comfortable as possible ... ... that helps you to relax ... ... you can close your eyes, so it becomes even more comfortable ... ...Let the music come into the room ... ... perceive it ... ... feel the rhythm ... ... and concentrate on the music as if you could hear words behind the melody ... ... and at the same time you do hear my voice ... ... Perhaps you have already noticed that my voice is almost the same Volume is like music ... ... But sometimes your perception changes, although I speak with the same volume ... ... Sometimes the music may come to you louder than my voice ... ... Then you hear the music more strongly and you have to listen to mine intensely Concentrate your voice ... ... Then again it can be different ... ... because you decide to hear my voice more clearly ... ... Then you concentrate, and my voice will clearer ... ... louder and easier to understand ... ... my voice is suddenly louder than the music ... ... So you concentrate on the music and on my voice ... ... maybe you have already noticed how quickly you come to rest inside ... ... The calm goes deeper and deeper ... ... how by itself ... ... through the music and through my voice ... ... you become calmer and calmer ... ..and exhale slowly and for a long time ... ... just like that ... ... Now concentrate on the feeling of the skin in your face ... ... maybe it is a little tense because you want to relax even more deeply ... ... just relax your face ... ... let go of all the muscles in your face and relax your face ... ... first the forehead ... ... then the eyes ... ... the cheeks ... ... and finally the Mouth and jaw ... ... Then watch the temperature in the room ... ... You can feel it on your face ... ... your scan tell you whether it is warm here or rather cool ... ... maybe also neutral ... ... or just pleasant ... ... perceive the feeling of the skin on your face clearly. .. ... Make yourself be aware of this feeling and let it become very clear ... ... Perhaps you have already noticed that your face becomes warmer if you concentrate fully on it... ... The more you manage to concentrate on your face, the deeper you go into the state of inner calm ... ... It's very easy ... ... it works by itself ... ... sinking deeper and deeper you in inner calm ... ... step by step ... ... you can feel the calm more and more clearly ... ...and maybe you want to become a lot calmer ... ... by focusing even more on the feeling......focus on the skin of your face ... ... your body adjusts itself more and more to rest and relaxation ... ... deeper and calmer ... ...

Introduction 2:

... ... Close your eyes and breathe in deeply and slowly and long out ... ... take another deep breath ... ... and exhale slowly and for a long time ... ... just like that ... ... Now concentrate on the feeling of the skin in our face ... ... is maybe a little tense because you want to relax even more deeply ... ... just relax your face ... ... let go of all things in the face and relax your face ... ... is the forehead ... ... then the eyes ... ... the cheeks ... ... and the cavity mouth and jaw... ... then watch the temperature in the room ... ... You can see it on your face ... ... yours Skin can be yours, whether it is warm here or rather cool ... ... possibly also neutral ... ... or just heard ... ... You can clearly perceive the feeling of the skin on your face. .. ... Make yourself be aware of this feeling and let it be very open ... ... You may have heard that your face will be warmer if you follow more direct guidelines...... The more you manage to belong on your face, the deeper you go into it State of inner calm ... ... it's very easy ... ... it goes by itself ... ... sinking deeper and deeper you in inner calm ... ... step by step ... ... you can feel the calm more and more clearly ... ... and maybe you want to be a lot calmer ... ... you compensate yourself even more for the feeling the skin of your face you see ... ... your body is more and more certain of rest and relaxation ... ... ever deeper and calmer ... ...

Introduction 3:

… … Make yourself comfortable now … … Find the position that feels best to be in a trance go … … take the blanket to make yourself even more comfortable … … snuggle up in it, if you want, maybe you'd rather go into a trance without a blanket … … do it like this, how it feels best … … close your eyes … … Now let your breathing become calm to relax even more deeply … … step by step … …at your speed … … at your pace … … it becomes calmer and calmer inside you … … with everyone second you relax a little deeper … … just adjust to the most beautiful and deepest relaxation that you can imagine … …with your eyes closed, just imagine how you just did that … … First you did you have found the best position to go into a trance and have already become calmer … …then you have used the wool blanket to make yourself even more comfortable and have yourself deeper relaxed … … when you closed your eyes you became even more calm … … with your breathing you could finally go deeper into a trance … … Now everything works by itself … … Your relaxation goes deeper with every breath … …

Deepening of trance 1:

... ... Now I will help you to relax more deeply ... ... The main thing is to calm down your body ... ... Maybe you knew that physical relaxation and inner peace Going hand in hand ... ... So when your body comes to rest, yours automatically rotates too Look inside ... ... and you will be calmer ... ... Perhaps you are wondering how best to do it is that your body can relax ... ... It's probably easier than you think ... ... yours The body can relax by making a wish ... ... if you now, for example wish that your shoulders should relax, then that happens too ... ... just wish you that your shoulders should relax ... ... Maybe you can already feel it ... ... Maybe too a little later ... ... just carry on ... ... Formulate the inner wish that your body should relax ... ... wish that your arms relax, your hands too, and of course also your fingers ... ... and with each relaxation of your body you go deeper into this wonderful inner peace ... ... just make a wish ... ... So tell your body, your upper body should now relax ... ... your stomach ... ... yours Back ... ... the spine ... ... and if you just wait a little, you will feel it too ... ... Everything relaxes because you do it that way want ... ... because it is your wish ... ... because it is your command to your body ... ... everything happens as you want it ... ... your legs should now relax ... ... the thighs ... ...the lower legs ... ... and also the feet should relax ... ... and you can in a pleasant rest ... ... deeper and deeper if you want it that way ... ..

Deepening of trance 2:

... ... Breathe calmly and evenly...... And now start counting...... It's very simple...... You start at 100 ... ... you just count backwards ... ... and you open for every odd number the eyes ... ... You close them again with every even number ... ... This is how you do one with every number eye movement ... ... just count and open your eyes, close your eyes ... ... open your eyes, close your eyes ... ... that is very simple ... ... If I ask you to start counting right away, you will just start to count ... ... so loud that I can hear you ... ... and I'll just talk to you ... ... but you keep counting ... ... start counting now ... ... start at 100 ... ...

... ... [we help the client's counting rhythm with the first numbers with the words "Open your eyes - close your eyes – eyes open - close your eyes ".] ... ...

... ... It can get exhausting over time...... Above all, always finding the right numbers...... Perhaps the numbers will soon be unimportant...... It then becomes more and more difficult and harder to find the right number ... ... And maybe soon you won't feel like anymore, to continue counting ... ... But you continue ... ...

... ... [eyes open - eyes closed - eyes open - eyes closed] ... ...

... ... Maybe you noticed that you just forgot a number ... ... It doesn't matter ... ... It just shows that you can relax well ... ... Numbers are then not so important ... ... Just keep trying if you want ... ... And if you want, you can relax too ... ... If it becomes too annoying for you, you can just go into a nice relaxation and stop counting ... ...

Deepening of trance 3:

… … First allow yourself some rest … … And then imagine a beautiful flower, the most beautiful that you have can imagine. Imagine it exactly and focus your inner gaze directly on this flower … … maybe your favorite flower … … maybe a flower that doesn't even exist … … choose a color for it … … and then always look at this flower … … only that is important now … … you always look at this flower … … directly at this flower … … and your gaze turns inward … … and you come to rest … … and step by step you can relax … …simply by looking at this flower … … always only at this one flower … … your gaze turns more and more inwards … … and you come to rest more and more … …Perhaps you can already feel the relaxation…… It is slowly developing in you…… and you still fix your gaze on that one flower … … you see the petals … … you recognize the color … … If you want, you can now step by step into a beautiful interior going to rest … … ever deeper and deeper … … as deep as you want … … and now even deeper in to go to relaxation, you can hide the image of the flower … …

Promotion of willingness to change (compliance) 1: For those affected

...... In the calm that you have now found, you fully adjust to your body constructively influence ...... you want to get healthy ...... as healthy as you can. ...... there is also a sensitive and fine body feeling helpful ...... In this moment you feel good and are relaxed ...... therefore you are also sensitive to your body ...... if you now look at your Paying attention to your breathing ...... paying all your attention to the rhythm of your breathing, then you can feel the movements of your body exactly ...... It rises and falls with every breath ...... Now, in your awareness, let exactly this movement step forward and make it you are aware of it ...... The more you concentrate on your breathing, the more clearly you feel also the movement of your body ...... So concentrate and feel your breath in and out flow ...... feel the rhythm of your body ...... you feel this rhythm much more clearly than usual ...... you feel your body much better and perceive it more consciously ...... Exactly now ...... that is the best basis for changing your body ...... conscious perception ...... like now ...... just like now ......

Promotion of willingness to change (compliance) 2: For those affected

...... Today you want to help your body to become healthy ...... want to activate its own deep power and let it become free ...... You know that to do this you first change your inner attitude have to ...... the inner attitude, the basic attitude that tells you: I will get well ...... is the right prerequisite to bring your body step by step into a constructive and wholesome state ...... to encourage and support him as far as possible and as soon as possible to get healthy as possible ...... To do this, you make it clear to yourself at this very moment that you have already found your inner attitude towards this, because that is exactly why you are here ...... you know them correct posture that tells you: I will get well! ......

...... You can take it even more, still go deeper into this posture to use it even better for you ......The strength that you need to go fully into this basic attitude and to stay in it lies deep within to yourself ...... deep in the calm that you feel now ...... So you immerse yourself completely in this inner calm and lets them become very conscious ...... The more you can feel the inner calm, the sooner you will become discover new strength ...... both are directly related ...... You feel calm and find your strength...... Concentrate again on the feeling of calm and thus open a door for the new one and intense power and strength deep inside you ...... just like that ......

Promotion of willingness to change (compliance) 3: For relatives

… … You have a goal … … You want the rigors of treatment together with your loved one … … *[better name or role … with your mother … with your girlfriend etc.]* … … wear him / her support … … and find strength for yourself again and again … … because you too have so that you can endure a lot of stresses that cost you strength … … you also need again and again Balance … … inner balance … … healing for you … … that was not always easy to achieve, but today it will be easier … … much easier than before … …Quiet is not always easy to find … … But right now, at this very moment, feel you are completely calm and relaxed inside … … and in fact you feel pretty It's easy to be so calm and relaxed by simply following the flow of relaxation you just let go, you let my voice lead and carry you … … you got it just let it happen … … It's that simple today … … It's that simple right now ……If such relaxation is easy today, then your goal is easier to achieve too … …As soon as you succeed in deepening your relaxation, you will also succeed in reaching your goal more quickly … … align yourself completely with your goal … … so relax just deeper … … you know how to do it … … you just did it … … do it so again and relax deeper … … the deeper you relax, the faster you reach your goal of losing weight and being slim … … so relax more deeply … …

Main Part 1: Persevering in Chemotherapy

Classic suggestion hypnosis (for those affected)

Classical suggestion depends on formulations that promote a constructive attitude and confirm the inner focus on the therapy goal. Various formulation techniques can be used here. The suggestions must be formulated in such a way that they are not interpreted as superficial and overly simple requests. It is therefore important to give the impression that the development described will occur naturally or has already occurred. Constructive formulations and small confirmations, which sometimes flow in very inconspicuously and almost casually, are helpful here. But don't be afraid of negations. As I always emphasize in many places in other books and in my seminars, it is a myth that the subconscious does not understand negations. The correct use of negative statements is decisive, because it must be suggested before, between the lines or after what should take place instead of the negative thought, feeling or behavior. It is also important to connect several processing levels that are in constant interaction with one another. I prefer the levels of thought, physicality, emotionality and behavior. The client is confronted with suggestions for change in all of these areas.

...... You often feel physically tired and burned out ...... powerless and drained ...... you feel how chemotherapy affects the body, causes nausea and exhaustion ...... maybe even pain sometimes ...... but you know that the treatment will help you ...... you have yourself therefore made to see it through ...... and it is really quite remarkable how much courage and strength you have already mustered to actually go through it all ...... Now it comes down to it to find peace and relaxation again so that your body can recover from the strenuous treatment ......let your breathing become conscious and breathe in and out consciously ...... very consciously ...... in ......and off ...... *[in the actual breathing rhythm of the client please]* ...... on ...... and off ...... if you once paying attention to your breath, you can clearly feel the air coming in and out through your nose flows out ...... with every breath ...... you can feel it ...... through breathing you can body now find rest ...... To do this, imagine that you are in your entire body could breathe into it ...... as if fresh air flows through your whole body with every breath flows ...... and when you breathe out it relaxes even more and becomes calmer ...... Let's start with your arms ...... Breathe in deeply and feel the air flowing into your arms ...... very deep ...... down to the fingertips ...... and when you breathe out, the air flows back again ......if there was still tension now, you could feel it because the air wouldn't flow unhindered ...... so if there is something left, you can let go of it with the exhale ...... And your arms become calmer ... This is how you do it with the next breaths ...... your arms relax more and more ...... the left arm ...... and also the right arm ...... Now to the head ...... Pay attention to your breath and direct it to the head ...... You can feel how the breath pulls through the nose to behind the eyes ...... The fresh air is distributed in your whole head ...... You can let go of everything that is disturbing you with the exhalation and afterwards lead outside...... thoughts or considerations...... doubts or fears...... With every breath your head relaxes...... deeper and deeper...... so your head becomes whole free and carefree ...... completely free and calm ...... with the next breaths, the air flows into your upper body ...... first into the lungs ...... and from there on into the muscles of the back and abdomen ...... into all internal organs ... ... Here, too, you would notice if there were obstacles ... ... if something was still tense should be, then you feel it and can dissolve it ... ... and when you breathe out you let go of it ... ...your upper body comes to rest ... ... You allow your upper body to experience rest ... ...as you continue to breathe in peace, your body relaxes more and more ... ... all parts of your body, which have already been mentioned, deepen the rest and relaxation ... ... with every breath ... ... with every single breath ... ...you're doing well ... ... It's just as right as you are doing it right now ... ... So your relaxes your body best and comes to new strength and strength ... ... And if you have forgotten something or have overlooked something ... ... then you can do it now in move your legs ... ... with a few breaths your whole upper body fills ... ... also your arms and your head with oxygen ... ... and when you breathe out any tension that might be gone has remained here and there, in your legs ... ... Now everything that could still be disturbing flows into yours legs............ You breathe in deeply, and the air flows very deep into your legs...... You breathe out and everything that somehow disturbs or pinches ... ... everything that is now still tense or cramped flows while over the soles of your feet to the outside ... ... With each exhalation you let go of tension and send them out over the soles of your feet and the tips of your toes ... ... and you'll be there calmer ... ... and your body comes to rest and relaxes completely ... ... more and more ... ... and more and more ... ... Well, it's exactly right ... ... You are doing the right thing, and it's very simple ... ... You just have to breathe in and out, that's enough ... ... *[in the rhythm of the client please]* ... ... on and off ... ... that's enough ... ... on and off ... ... that's enough ... ...now you can enjoy the relaxation...... You feel how relaxed your body feels...... maybe as relaxed as it has not been for a long time...... And maybe are you asking yourself if you can give your body even more rest ... ... if it is possible, right now to relax even deeper now and give your body some rest ... ... Then you just breathe more ... ... Every breath helps you ... ... Every breath gently caresses your body ... ... Now you will surely also feel how good it is when you create this calm state for your body ... ... how relaxing it is ... ... you feel it more and more clearly and at the same time see how simply it is ... ... your body finds strength and courage again ... ... hope and strength ... ... balance and healing power ... ... new healing power ... ...

Consolidation (post-hypnotic assignment)

... ... But every day your body can and may recover ... ... regenerate from all the stresses ... ... You can help him, just like today ...... just like now .... You just make yourself comfortable every day for a while ...... as comfortable as you can, also and especially then, if you are feeling sick or in pain ...... You find a while every day of peace, ... and your breathing will help you find peace and calm even deeper and your body to purify ...... to find new strength ...... new freshness ...... vitality and strength ...... exactly like that like now and maybe even more ...... because your deep inside learns better every time, how it can take the path of rest and renewal ... your deep inside learns with each time better how it can help you regenerate your body ...... help it get healthy ... ...

Main part 2: Accompany chemotherapy

Classic suggestion hypnosis (for relatives)

Classical suggestion depends on formulations that promote a constructive attitude and confirm the inner focus on the therapy goal. Various formulation techniques can be used here. The suggestions must be formulated in such a way that they are not interpreted as superficial and overly simple requests. It is therefore important to give the impression that the development described will occur naturally or has already occurred. Constructive formulations and small confirmations, which sometimes flow in very inconspicuously and almost casually, are helpful here. But don't be afraid of negations. As I always emphasize in many places in other books and in my seminars, it is a myth that the subconscious does not understand negations. The correct use of negative statements is decisive, because it must be suggested before, between the lines or after what should take place instead of the negative thought, feeling or behavior. It is also important to connect several processing levels that are in constant interaction with one another. I prefer the levels of thought, physicality, emotionality and behavior. The client is confronted with suggestions for change in all of these areas.

... ... Chemotherapy is exhausting and dangerous treatment ... ... But it is not only then Stress, if you were affected by it yourself ... ... You know what it is like to accompany a loved one in getting through chemotherapy ... ... That's a stress for you too ... ... because you are worried about how things will continue ... ... because you don't have the disease yourself can influence and sometimes have the feeling of having to watch helplessly and wait ... ... Then you have a lot of thoughts ... ... So you also need a way to come to terms with all this, to become lighter and to let go of burdens again and again ... ... You too want to be healthy and stay healthy ... ... and you have every right in this world to do so ... ...Today you can concentrate completely on yourself...... Today it should only be about you and your health is going ... ... Maybe you think that you are already healthy ... ... Yes Health is more than the absence of illness ... ... health means joy of life ... ... Strength ... ... hope ... ... you can be healthy and feel good ... ... so you start with to allow yourself to feel good ... ... even and especially if it is a loved one If things go bad, you have to be allowed to feel good, because only healthy and strong can you muster the strength to help him / her ... ... It's really amazing how well you are doing at this moment, you to allow yourself to be healthy once ... ... with a clear conscience ... ... This is exactly what you concentrate more and more on ... ... on your good conscience, because that is exactly what you are entitled to ... ...Allow yourself once again very clearly to be healthy and even more, to feel good ... ... you can feel good ... ... Enjoy this moment in which you can feel really good ... ... right now ... ... right here ... ... exactly like this ... ... If you listen deeply into yourself, you will feel that you have become tired yourself...... that yours Body sends signals of exhaustion...... So next you concentrate on your body feeling ... ... Today you allow your body to relax very intensely...... to rest and in the process to come to new strength ... ... It is remarkable how well you manage your body to send this signal ... ... to allow your body to finally come to rest now ... ... because that's exactly what helps you to stay healthy ... ... stronger and more self-confident ... ... and with it Much healthier ... ... The more you manage to be and stay healthy yourself, the better can you actually do for your sick relatives ... ... *[Please add here who it is acts ... for your sick mother ... ...]* ... ... to be there ... ... always give yourself and your body a gift more mindfulness and love ... ... mindfulness and love ... ... just like that ... ... With every breath your mindfulness becomes more intense ... ... the mindfulness of you for you ... ... more intensely with every single breath ... ... So pay close attention to your breath and let it go to flow very consciously ... ... Follow the pull of your breath and show your body that you are Allowing him rest and health ... ... It is great how well you manage to help yourself and your body to finally come to rest and find new strength ... ... new health for you ... ... because that's exactly what you deserve ... ... Breathe calmly and evenly ... ... just like that ... just like that ... ... Then you deal with your feelings of guilt ... ... You often have this strange one Feeling that healthy people often have when a relative gets sick ... ... the healthy ones People then feel uncomfortable and secretly guilty because they are allowed to be healthy themselves ... ... But this thinking is a mistake ... ... We can all get healthy ... ... be healthy ... ... and stay healthy ... ... we have good wishes for our sick ... ... prayers and hopes ... ...We don't know when they can be healthy again ... ... But you can be healthy with a clear conscience ... ... healthy with a clear conscience ... ... now in this calm ... ... here and today ...... at this very moment you can see it that way ... ... you can see that you are innocent ... ... you can now let go of your feelings of guilt ... ... You can do just that now ... ... you let go of all negative thoughts ... ... you let go of every bad conscience ... ... you let go of everyone Feel free to guilt ... ... because that's the way it is ... ... that's how it should be ... ... free from guilt and healthy ... ... and with every breath the feeling of inner freedom becomes bigger and clearer ... ... with every single breath it becomes clearer to you and this thought becomes more stable: I am innocent ... ... I am innocent ... ... With every breath you can hear it deep inside you like your own voice ... ... I am innocent ... ... I am innocent ... ... With every breath the feeling of inner freedom more intense ... ... freedom from all guilt ... ... with every single breath more intensely ... ... So pay close attention to your breath and let it flow very consciously ... ... Follow that

Take your breath and hear your inner voice that says: I am innocent ... ... Yes, I am and remain without guilt ... ... I am free...... I am free...... It is remarkable how well you manage to hear your inner voice and to accept its words ... ... Very remarkable, how good you are now can help yourself by being important to yourself and taking care of yourself ... ... you today and keep thinking about your self-awareness ... ...

Consolidation (post-hypnotic assignment)

... ... My words and the words of your inner voice are deeply anchored in your subconscious ... ...Everything is deeply impressed in your feelings ... ... So you can every day, if you want, breathe in a very targeted way for letting go and breathe for your inner freedom ... ... Whenever you are completely Breathe out consciously and deliberately slowly and for a long time, because you want to let go, you immediately feel the inner one Liberation ... ... becoming lighter ... ... you simply exhale slowly and long in a targeted manner and feel your letting go ... ... Whenever you have the feeling that old thoughts might come back, you just breathe out slowly and long ... ... slowly and long ... ... and let go let's go ... ... just like today ... ... just like today ... ... In this way you will always find strength to support your loved ones ... ... *[please insert the person being looked after or affected]* ... ... to continue his recovery accompany ... ... continue to bear the stresses of chemo together with him / her ... ...

Main part 3: activate self-healing power

Anchor technology (for those affected)

The following hypnosis session works with a symbolic anchor. One calls an anchor a trigger that can create a certain feeling or arouse a certain thought should. We want to help the client, by holding a hand flatterer, the feeling of a strong self-healing power in the form of great trust in one's own deep-seated powers to call consciousness. To do this, it is necessary to first establish a state in which the Client in trance consciously experiences self-confidence and positive thoughts. This feeling will then associated and anchored with the grasping and holding of a hand flatterer. Subsequently in phases of despair and discouragement, the client should be able to use this hand flatterer as an aid to get back into a state of hope and despair as quickly as possible Trust to arrive. Any hand flatterer that the client likes or agrees with can be used, also a healing stone. It always depends on the balance between realistic healing prospects and forward-looking thoughts of healing Find. On the one hand, hope and belief in healing should be more optimistic than the prognosis, in order to really get to the self-healing potential of the organism that not is accessible to the mind. On the other hand, the gap between suggestion and imaginable healing should not become implausible; otherwise the effect of hypnosis is quickly lost. To put it very directly: Although there are also "miraculous healings", it makes no sense in hypnotized to claim that stray cancer will soon go away if only the thoughts are positive enough. Overall, psychotherapeutic treatment of cancer is primarily about dealing with the disease and the changes it is having in the client's life brings himself to deal with. This is more important than healing suggestions. At the same time, my experience shows that believers in self-healing powers and deep-seated energies of the organism often makes an essential contribution to recovery, both for the inner attitude towards the treatment and recovery process as well as for the actual question of the healing prospects. With this, as with all hypnoses in the book, please note that there is always an individual adjustment to the specific illness and condition of the client.

… … I will now help you to really activate your own self-healing power … … it can help you to make as clear progress as possible in recovery … … What we call self-healing power can also help you to get through difficult phases of treatment more easily, to find hope and trust again and again … …strength for the next Steps … …To this end, today we will jointly strengthen the self-healing power of your organism ……… But first you can make yourself really comfortable, now find peace … … you will. Inwardly more and more calm and concentrate only on the feeling of calm … … After all the stresses and strains, you now deserve rest … … Sink deeper and deeper into a wonderful trance … … deeper and deeper … … with every word that I say you go a little deeper in this beautiful state of inner calm … … you're doing it right, you just allow it, just let it happen and drift all by yourself, at your own pace, at your own pace in this beautiful state of deep … … inner … … calm … … good so … … very good ……Now feel deep inside you the trust in yourself … … Your deep trust is waiting deep inside you and can get stronger … … sink deeper and deeper and find your trust in yourself … … so You have already experienced and endured a lot, because only your trust in you and your strength has this enables you … … the more you manage to get into a calm state, the more you feel this trust … … and you are already in a calm state, so you have already found the trust … … maybe without noticing it, but it is here … … deep in you … … let this trust become more and more evident, because you need it now … … it is here …… deep inside you … … let this trust become even stronger, because you need it now … … itis here … … deep within you … … you have found it … … excellent … … because if you have found it, and you have, then it becomes clearer at precisely this moment … … at this very moment … … good so … … very, very good so … …It is this inner trust that helps you … … It helps you get through difficult times … It helps you to be strong and to recover quickly … … It helps you to have the greatest possible strength in you awaken and use … … your inner self-healing power … … the power of your organism, yourself to heal yourself as well and as far as possible lies in precisely this inner trust … … you can use it very particularly today, because now she is in a state of inner calm, in a trance more freely and can move unhindered ... ... Now your organism helps you to heal your Illness particularly intense ... ... The more you trust yourself or simply if you concentrate on the idea of trust, the more your organism can now help with healing ... ...I will now give you the flatterer in the hand ... ... *[Name the symbol actually used ... the healing stone... the wooden lion etc.]* ... ... take it and hold it tight ... ... it should be your healing anchor ... ...that's right ... ... Hold on to your healing anchor and at the same time feel the trust deep within you...... Both become one...... your healing anchor and your trust...... This is how both work together...... Because whenever you feel your healing anchor in your hand, it immediately becomes your deep one trust awake and help you with all your inner power of self-healing ... ... now and every time, when you take the healing anchor in your hand, you feel your inner trust very strongly ... ... like now, even more clearly ... ...

Consolidation (post-hypnotic assignment)

... ... Hold the healing anchor tight now ... ... Concentrate on the feeling in your hand ... ... this feeling shows you now and in the future that your organism has all the power to heal itself ... ... You will feel even more trust and confidence ... ... every day you can activate and strengthen this trust and also the power of healing by taking the healing anchor, your personal healing anchor, in your hand and feeling it with your eyes closed ...... You can move it in your hand, feel it...... or you can hold it and press it... ... do it the way it feels best ... ... just take your healing anchor every day in your hand and feel it and your organism immediately provides trust and healing power ... ... trust and healing power ... ... just like now ... ... just like now ... ... hold your healing anchor firmly so that it connects even more with you ... ... with your healing power ... ...

... ... *[Continue the transition and let the client hold the healing anchor until hold the end of the session.]* ... ...

Forwarding, publication & copying in any form is prohibited and subject to compensation.

Copying, publishing and passing on to third parties is prohibited and only permitted with the written consent of the author Ingo Simon. Please carefully observe the information on copyright and use.

Main part 4: activate self-healing power

Anchor technology (for relatives)

The following hypnosis session works with a symbolic anchor. One calls an anchor a trigger that can create a certain feeling or arouse a certain thought should. We want to help the client, by holding a hand flatterer, the feeling of a strong self-healing power in the form of great trust in one's own deep-seated powers to call consciousness. To do this, it is necessary to first establish a state in which the Client in trance consciously experiences self-confidence and positive thoughts. This feeling will then associated and anchored with the grasping and holding of a hand flatterer. Subsequently in phases of despair and discouragement, the client should be able to use this hand flatterer as an aid to get back into a state of hope and despair as quickly as possible Trust to arrive. Any hand flatterer that the client likes or agrees with can be used, also a healing stone. It always depends on the balance between realistic healing prospects and forward-looking thoughts of healing Find. On the one hand, hope and belief in healing should be more optimistic than the prognosis, in order to really get to the self-healing potential of the organism that not is accessible to the mind. On the other hand, the gap between suggestion and imaginable healing should not become implausible; otherwise the effect of hypnosis is quickly lost. To put it very directly: Although there are also "miraculous healings", it makes no sense in hypnotized to claim that stray cancer will soon go away if only the thoughts are positive enough. Overall, psychotherapeutic treatment of cancer is primarily about dealing with the disease and the changes it is having in the client's life brings himself to deal with. This is more important than healing suggestions. At the same time, my experience shows that believers in self-healing powers and deep-seated energies of the organism often makes an essential contribution to recovery, both for the inner attitude towards the treatment and recovery process as well as for the actual question of the healing prospects. With this, as with all hypnoses in the book, please note that there is always an individual adjustment to the specific illness and condition of the client.

… … I will now help you to really activate your own self-healing power … … it can help you to regain a balanced mental state in order to be healthy stay … … and if you feel sick or attacked yourself, maybe exhausted and drained, then your inner strength will help you to become completely healthy and strong again … …what we call self-healing power can also help you through difficult phases of treatment of your dear relatives … … [better name … your son … your father etc.] … … easier to get through, to find hope and trust again and again … … strength for the next steps … … Today we will strengthen the self-healing power of your organism together … …First, however, you can make yourself really comfortable, now find peace … … You become more and calmer inside and only concentrate on the feeling of calm … … After all the stresses and strains and effort you deserve rest now…… Sink deeper and deeper into a wonderful trance…… Deeper and deeper…… with every word I say, you go a little deeper into this wonderful state of inner calm…… You are doing it right, you just let it happen, you just let it happen and drive all by itself, at your speed, at your own pace in these beautiful state of deep … … inner … … calm … … good so … … very good … … …Now feel deep inside you the trust in yourself … … Your deep trust is waiting deep inside you and can get stronger … … sink deeper and deeper and find your trust in yourself … … so you have already experienced and endured a lot, because only your trust in you and your strength has this enables you … … you know many difficult phases in your own life … … maybe also serious illnesses … … and also the accompaniment of your loved one … … [better concrete name … your son … your father etc.] … … is a difficult time for you, in which you too have strength have left and can use help … … The more you manage to get into a calm state, the more you will feel this too trust in you that can help you to get through all of this … … and be in a calm state you do, so you've already found confidence … … maybe without noticing it, but it is here … … deep within you … … let this trust become clearer and clearer, because you need it now … … it is here … … deep within you … … let this trust become even stronger, because you need it now … … it is here … … deep inside you … … you found it … … out outstanding ... ... because when you have found it, and you have it, then it will be exactly in this one Moment clearer ... ... exactly at this moment ... ... good that way ... ... very, very good that way ... ... It is this inner trust that helps you ... ... It helps you get through difficult times ... It helps you to be strong and to recover quickly ... ... It helps you to have the greatest possible strength in you awaken and use ... ... your inner self-healing power ... ... the power of your organism, yourself Balancing or healing yourself as well and as much as possible over and over again is exactly what you need this inner trust ... ... You can use it very particularly today, because now in the state of inner peace, in a trance, she is freer and can move unhindered ... ... Now yours will help you Organism is particularly intense in healing your illness ... ... The more you focus on that Trust or just focus on the idea of trust, all the more it can help your organism to heal now ... ... I will now give you the flatterer in the hand ... ... *[Name the symbol actually used ... the healing stone ... the wooden lion etc.]* ... ... take it and hold it tight ... ... it should be your anchor of strength ... ... That's right ... ... hold on to your power anchor and at the same time feel the trust deep inside you ... ... Both become one ... ... your anchor of strength and your trust ... ... This is how both work together...... Because whenever you feel your power anchor in your hand, your deep trust immediately becomes awake and helps you with all your inner power of self-healing ... ... now and every time you take the healing anchor in your hand, you feel your inner trust very strongly ... ... like now, even more clearly ... ...

Consolidation (post-hypnotic assignment)

... ... Hold the power anchor tight now ... ... Concentrate on the feeling in your hand ... ... this feeling shows you now and in the future that your organism has all the power to heal itself ... ... So you feel even more trust and confidence ... ... Every day you can activate and strengthen this trust and also the power of healing by using the power anchor, take your personal power anchor in your hand and feel it with your eyes closed ...

... You can move it in your hand, feel it ... ... or you can hold it and press it ... ... Do it the way it feels best ... ... just put your power anchor in your hand every Hand and feel it and immediately your organism provides trust and healing power ... ... trust and healing power ... ... like now ... ... just like now ... ... hold on to your power anchor so that it connects even more with you ... ... with your healing power ... ...

... ... *[Continue the transition and let the client hold the healing anchor until hold the end of the session.]* ... ...

Main Part 5: Soap Bubbles against Cancer

Creative Association (for those affected)

The following hypnosis text works with creative association. That means a scene or an image is selected that is understood as a symbol for the topic to be treated and so stands as a proxy for the problem. The change and realignment of the scene or of the picture then leads in a second step to a change in the problem view and opening for new ways. Here rules of suggestion are less important than imagination and inner creativity of the client. The pictures are therefore partly offered with many details; on the other hand, a lot is deliberately left open. This approach is a Cooperative type of hypnosis that relies on inner self-development in the state of trance and therefore leads much less than suggestion hypnosis.

… … You know cancer well by now. You also know the difficult fight against … … you know that it helps you to stand up against it … … Sometimes you may also wish the sick ones to be able to simply let go of the cells of your body … … as if you could throw them overboard or spit out … … Then your thoughts circle around the question of why it hit you in particular … … Sometimes you might have thought that the illness was like a punishment … … Yes then again you realize that there are no such punishments … … All these probing thoughts burden you very much, perhaps more than you realize … … because you have so much to do with the disease do … … are constantly confronted with cancer, so that there is no other way than your thoughts to deal with it … … But today something else should happen … … Today it should be about to let go of all disturbing thoughts once … … these thoughts that tend to be slow in healing do … … As soon as you manage to let go of the disturbing thoughts, your organism can concentrate even better on the healing … … and you will feel more comfortable … … This requires that you change your thoughts and feelings … … So you want to Let go of those disturbing thoughts and feelings … … Maybe you are already excited to see how that works … … You imagine that every single thought is a small colored ball that is in your head … … All feelings are also located as small balls in your head … … so you just have to find the disturbing thoughts and feelings to let go of them … … you can recognize them by their color … … your breathing will help you … … For example, let's take a look at your depressed mood … … your tiredness and severity … … your inner depression … … So you can imagine that all thoughts and all feelings that belong to your depressed mood, the color blue … … *[The colors can of course be exchanged; they are chosen arbitrarily and are filled with suggestions.]* … … carry … … So there are a lot of little blue balls in your head that you can let go of … … …You do this with your breathing … … you breathe in and the air you breathe flows through your head … … You can see it in your inner eye … … The air you breathe collects all blue thoughts and feelings and carry them with you … … And you breathe them out … … … They come out of yours as soap bubbles nose and float through the room ... ... Lots of blue soap bubbles ... ... And one after the other dissolves ... ... they just burst ... ... and you carry on ... ... you inhale and collect all blue thoughts and feelings in ... ... you breathe them out like soap bubbles ... ... they float through the room and dissolve ... ... You repeat that with every breath. Your depressed mood is dissolving more and more ... ... You're deep inside is now leaving new thoughts arise ... ... You feel the feeling of hope ... ... It works by itself. You just keep breathing and watch the blue soap bubbles that ... ... Now let's look at your feelings of guilt ... ... because you have often accused yourself ... ... you may even now think that you did something wrong or that you were to blame and that's why you got sick ... ... All thoughts and feelings with guilt are connected are yellow ... ... So there are a lot of yellow balls in your head that you let go ... ... you breathe in and collect all the yellow thoughts and feelings ... ... and you breathe them out ... ... They come out of your nose as soap bubbles and float through the room ... ... Lots of yellow soap bubbles ... ... And one after the other dissolves ... ... They just burst ... ... And you go on ... ... you breathe in and collect all the yellow thoughts and feelings ... ... You breathe them out as soap bubbles ... ... They float through the room and dissolve ... ... That you repeat with every breath ... ... Your deep inner being lets new thoughts arise again. You become free and you realize that you are innocent ... ... It works by itself ... ... You just keep breathing and watch the yellow soap bubbles dissolve ... ... you are innocent ... ... you are and always will be innocent ... ... Next up is your perfectionism ... ... you know how it is ... ... you have so often tries to do everything particularly well ... ... to do everything better and better and not fail to have ... ... Also in the fight against your illness you gave everything again and again ... ... Perhaps there were times of desperation, but you kept pulling yourself up and moving on done ... ... All thoughts and feelings that deal with perfectionism or lead to perfectionism are red ... ... So there are a lot of red balls in your head that you let go of can ... ... you breathe in and collect all the red thoughts and feelings ... ... and you breathe them from ... ... They come out of your nose as soap bubbles and float through the room ... ... Louder red soap bubbles ... ... and one by one dissolves ... ... they just burst ... ... and you carry on ... ... you breathe in and collect all the red thoughts and feelings ... ... as soaps you breathe them out ... ... they float through the room and dissolve .. ... Repeat that with every breath ... ... your deep inner being lets new thoughts arise again. To the Instead of perfectionism comes serenity and consideration for yourself ... ... This is how by itself ... ... you just keep breathing and watch the red soap bubbles dissolve ... ... Serenity and consideration become stronger ... ... Serenity and consideration become stronger ... ...

Consolidation (post-hypnotic assignment)

... ... Your deep inner being impresses everything ... ... Deep down you know that you can actually breathe out all disturbing thoughts and feelings, today and every day in your life ... ... You also know that everything you let go of will be replaced by new, helping, constructive thoughts ... ... so you will freer and stronger ... ... so you have more strength for your recovery ... ... today you can you feel it ... ... So you can feel it every other day in your life ... ... whenever you want, you just close your eyes for a moment and breathe out everything that is disturbing as colored soap bubbles ... ... Just like today, they burst and dissolve ... ... just like today ... ... And you feel new strength ... ...

Main part 6: Addressing the body

Creative Association (for those affected)

The following hypnosis text works with creative association. That means a scene or an image is selected that is understood as a symbol for the topic to be treated and so stands as a proxy for the problem. The change and realignment of the scene or of the picture then leads in a second step to a change in the problem view and opening for new ways. Here rules of suggestion are less important than imagination and inner creativity of the client. The pictures are therefore partly offered with many details; on the other hand, a lot is deliberately left open. This approach is a Cooperative type of hypnosis that relies on inner self-development in the state of trance and therefore leads much less than suggestion hypnosis.

... ... You know what it's like to have a body that doesn't always work properly ... ... you know them days when it is not easy to get physically healthy ... ... And now you want that with everyone strength ... ...get physically healthy again ... ... as healthy as it can be ... ... as pain-free and flexible as possible ... ... Today you will find a helping hand deep inside you power ... ... a power that will help you to strengthen your body as much as possible... ... a force that can help you heal ... ... a force in you that can contribute to it can help you get well again ... ... as good as possible ... ... Maybe you know that yourself in difficult and even in seemingly hopeless situations, more is still possible than the mind can imagine ... ... more than the mind often wants to believe ... ... that's why you are here today ... ... because deep down you believe that everything is possible, what you imagine or you can simply wish ... ... To this end, you focus your mindfulness on the helping side today of your body, because there are also...... So today you are talking to your body...... you go into this direct contact and focus your mindfulness on everything that your body already has did for you when he was still healthy and many parts of your body are still ... ... you thank your body today for everything that has worked well until today ... ... Also for the fact that he can and will help you to become healthier ... ... First you address yourself to your hands. You say thank you that she always grabbed it have ... ... they have often held on ... ... often let go ... ... they do their vigorous service every day, as best they can ... ... they can also give you hints as to when it is better to let go should ... ... because when you let go your hands become free again and open to new things ... ... Eighth on the feeling in your hands ... ... they signal to you when you can also let go internally ... ... Also that which could make you sick or contributed to your illness ... ... Let get rid of it now and free yourself from it ... ... *[what feels like a half-minute break]* ... ... Then speak with your arms ... ... they hold your hands and lift loads ... ... you know how it is difficult to bear loads, internally and externally ... ... always have your arms with you helped ... ... you thank them now, and they will continue to help you ... ... because it is theirs task to lend a hand for you ... ... to access when opportunities arise ... ... to do that carry what you want to hold and finally let go of what you do with your hands you no longer need ... ... Next you turn to your back ... ... It carries a lot of burdens ...... It also keeps your body upright and straight ... ... Your back has been so often done good offices for you ... ... worked well all these years and never complained ... ... sometimes was he bent over from all the burden ... ... She pushed you down so that you couldn't follow could look in front ... ... but your back has always helped you to straighten up to be able to look forward again ... ... and to go on powerfully ... ... you thank your back today for his faithful service that he has done all these years until today ... ... Then speak you with the internal organs ... ... you thank them for having done their work so well so often ... ... the interaction of all organs makes life possible. And every organ has always tries to make the best possible contribution ... ... every healthy thing still does it today and even organs that have become sick continue to work for us ... ... as best they can ... ... they work like a chain and pull together ... ... But sometimes a chain breaks or can no longer work as hard because a chain link has become weaker ... ... but all of them other organs try to keep the internal functioning of the organism upright ... ... they do the same weakens out as best they can ... ... Your organs have also been doing this for many years ... ... until today they do it ... ... Then you direct yourself to your heart ... ... It keeps pumping blood into it body and supplies all organs with oxygen and life ... ... It brings the oxygen and all that nutrients in the blood in all muscles like fuel in an engine ... ... It keeps beating ... ... every second of your life ... ... day and night ... ... you thank your heart that it all has struck the years for you, without a break ... ... in quiet, but also in stormy moments ... ... It always works and only rests in the small breaks between the beats ... ... yours source of life ... ... You then focus your mindfulness on your legs ... ... You say thank you to them for carrying your body for so long ... ... they carry the body, hold it upright and take you from one place to another ... ... they can move you, but can also stop to pause and linger, because that is also important and necessary ... ... but you also helped to be faster ... ... to overtake ... ... they accompany you faithfully and to help ... ... companions in the truest sense of the word ... ... After all, you address yourself to your skin ... ... Today you thank your skin ... ... for it, that she gave you protection and warmth ... ... for protecting the bones and the insides from attack ... ... for taking up dirt and washing it off again, so that your insides remain clean and clear ... ...

Consolidation (post-hypnotic assignment)

... ... Now turn to the sick spot or the sick area of your body ... ... concentrate focus on the diseased organ or the diseased area of your body ... ... remember how long too this area of your body was healthy and try to say thank you for the time as your whole body was still healthy ... ... You will succeed, because you know that it will help you find your peace to do with your body ... ... Now you allow yourself some rest ... ... You let your body rest and trust in its help...... You also tell your body to help...... you makes a pact with all your body parts ... ... you assure your body that you will take care of it carefully and that it will always have rest to recover from the rigors of treatment you give ... ... in return, your body tries to become healthier and stronger as quickly as possible ... ... that should be your pact ... ...

Main part 7: activate self-healing power

Ide motoric skills (for those affected)

The following hypnosis session works with the classic arm levitation (floating arm). With the help of suggestions or images, the arm levitation gives the impression that the body of the client can be moved without his involvement. The required muscle contraction is performed unconsciously, expressed somewhat imprecisely but understandably: the subconscious the client makes the movement that appears to the client to be controlled by others. Levitations increase belief in the special effects of hypnosis and show the client that it is gives more than what he actively decides and can consciously and deliberately influence. It is important that the client can observe the floating and then cataleptically (rigid) arm himself with his or her eyes. So always leave that with arm levitations and catalepsies open your eyes to see the result. Many clients otherwise believe that the entire Arm movement was just an illusion, some feel the movement when closed Eyes not very clear either. Don't worry, when you open your eyes you won't lose your trance and your catalepsy will remain stable! The stronger a sick person's own belief in them the more positive the treatment progress is, the more self-healing power of his organism is Cancer as well as all other diseases. Of course, hypnosis is not a miracle. So never promise a certain success (by the way, this is forbidden for all therapists anyway).

... ... I will now help you to really activate your own self-healing power ... ... it can help you help make the most significant progress possible in recovery ... ... We will today strengthen the self-healing power of your organism together ... ...

... ... [Now follows arm levitation, for which there are numerous possibilities. You will be the following not being able to read the text easily. At least you should go to the next section "Catalepsy" skips over when the arm has already risen far up so that the elbow is away from the Underlay takes off. If the proposed text is not sufficient, extend it or repeat it him until the arm goes up. If you put persuasiveness and emphasis in your voice, it will be quite easy.] ... ...

Levitation phase

... ... Take a look at your right arm and imagine that a big red balloon is tied to it ... ... with a string around your wrist ... ... The balloon is filled with a very light gas, so that it rises ... ... The balloon rises into the air and pulls your arm up with it ... ... Imagine this huge red balloon and watch it go ... ... it rises higher and higher and pulls your arm up ... ... Your arm follows the balloon and rises higher and higher ... ... your arm becomes light as a feather and just rises up ... ... leave it just happen and be happy about it ... ... A huge red balloon takes your arm with it up ... ... Your arm rises higher and higher ... ... It gets lighter and lighter and rises into the air ... ... Your arm rises higher and higher ... ... higher and higher ... ... just like that ... ... just like that ... ... outstanding ... ... your arm is light as a feather and rises all by itself, all by itself ... ... So it's easy ... ... Your arm rises higher and higher ... ... higher and higher ... ... Look at the balloon afterwards ... ... the balloon rises in the air and pulls your arm with it ... ... it pulls and pulls ... ... he pulls and pulls on your arm ... ... pulls and pulls ... ...

Catalepsy phase

… … And now your arm becomes completely rigid and firm … … *[emphasis on the voice]* … … your arm becomes held exactly like that, it stays in exactly this position … … your arm is light as a feather and absolutely firm … … He is immobile … … absolutely immobile … … Nothing and nobody can hold your arm now still move … … it remains rigid and firm and light as a feather … … as firm as an iron bar … … just like that … … that's right … … you can even look at your arm, you can look at it, he remains in exactly this position … … Now open your eyes and look at your arm, the remains in exactly this position … … now! … … *[If the eyes are not opened, please help a little. Consists in a deep trance little motivation to open their eyes, and it is also difficult for the client because he is very is tired. Help something like this … You can open your eyes, you can. So go ahead, open your eyes now and look at your arm! …]* … … Now close your eyes again and sink into a deep trance … … Your subconscious becomes you help now, it has already helped you because it has raised your arm for you and is now holding it still firm … … Now your subconscious will help you, your self-healing power to make you stronger and to make as much of it available to you as possible … … your arm will immediately flexible again and your subconscious provides you with the greatest possible self-healing power … …

Consolidation (post-hypnotic assignment)

… … Your arm is now flexible again and sinks very slowly onto the surface, your subconscious activates your self-healing power … … Your arm now slowly sinks back down … … very slowly … … and as soon as it arrives on the mat, you have self-healing power your organism is fully available … … This activation only lasts as long as yours arm needed to reach the surface … … Your arm sinks down at exactly the speed that your subconscious needs to optimally increase your self-healing power and to make it available to you … … and as soon as he touches the surface, your self-healing power is fully available and helps you with your recovery ... ... your arm slowly sinks onto the seat ... ...

... ... *[Keep on making suggestions until the arm reaches the surface. Then please solve ide motor / catalepsy with the following suggestion on]* ... ...

... ... Your arm is now completely mobile and under your control. Move your arm and your hand and check that you actually have full control over your body

Main Part 8: Mindfulness and Healing

Somatic-emotional therapy (for those affected)

The following hypnosis works with the connection of emotion and body. Since all feeling just like thoughts that show in physical reactions, sometimes clearly, often very discreetly, can be done with the help of focusing on body perceptions and attentive attention problem-solving can be worked on using the signals of the body. The client should be deeply be able to physically feel lying feelings and thus be able to react more quickly to signs of emotional change. Suggestive techniques help to get over an influencing of the to change body sensations also emotions, because not only do the feelings generate body reactions, targeted use of the body also affects the sensations. Joy, for example, creates a smile; conversely, an intentional smile also tends to lighten it the inner mood.

… … You have dealt extensively with all the things that can have contributed to your illness … … it there were physical reasons for it and physical conditions … … but you also know that there are psychological conditions that contribute to your illness … … how it works, how well yours The prognosis can be … … You have long since realized that your illness has a very high proportion psychological factors mean that you have to deal with your thoughts and feelings if you not only get healthy, but also stay healthy in the long term want … … and that's exactly what you want … … get healthy and then stay healthy … … you want it more than ever before … … get healthy and stay healthy … … So now concentrate on the area or part of your body that is affected by the disease most affected is…… Put all your attention on this area as if it were there just this one part of your body … … if you want, you can look at your body from the outside, as if you were standing next to you and could look at your body … … take this Now focus entirely on the area or area of your body affected by the disease your attention … … and give yourself mindfulness and care … … mindfulness and care … … Perhaps you are also wondering how that works, yourself or your body To be mindful … … It's very simple … … Just be there … … Just think of yours Body and stay with your thoughts with him … … Nothing else is important now … … That is enough … … Mindfulness is loving attention to the thoughts … … and that is very much more than we usually have left for ourselves … … we often turn to others, that do you know well … … so now turn to yourself and give yourself attention and loving thoughts … … …… Go with all your conscious thoughts to the place of your illness and feel there into it … … direct all of your mindfulness there … … Imagine a red dot on yours Body in front of the sick spot … … as if this spot was marked so that you can always put it in the Can take a look … … feel into your body, at precisely this point and sink into this point of your body … … dive with your attention there … … always leave it get darker … … sink in deeper and deeper … … ever deeper and deeper … … it gets darker and darker … … your thoughts get quieter and slowly fade into the background … … your thoughts fade into the background, because now comes it just depends on your feeling ... ... that feeling that sits so deep in your body, at the point of your illness ... ... much deeper than the body can feel ... ... very deep in the emotions ... behind the sick part of your body you will find a special feeling that is now becoming increasingly clear will...... let this feeling become conscious, however it may be...... however it is may feel ... ... It is the feeling that is behind and in your illness. This feeling you can now clearly see ... ... Do not judge it, because feelings are neither good nor bad ...... Feelings are an expression of our inner experiences and experiences...... of ours reactions to our living conditions and events ... ... Exactly this feeling, that behind the red dot is now becoming increasingly clear, can help you to get well again ... ... Exactly this feeling can help you to free yourself from thoughts that make you sick, so that your organism gets stronger for your recovery ... ... you let the feeling go ... ... you just let it become conscious so that you can decouple it from the illness ... ... you can also feel the feeling even without illness ... You can feel this feeling now ... ... and you can let it become clearer ... ... clearer ... ... more consciously ... ... let it become very intense, however it may be may feel ... ... It did not cause your illness, but it did contribute to it ... ... It slows down the healing ... ... But today everything will be different ... ... Today you recognize the feeling ... ... Today you free it and thus uncouple it from you and an illness ... ... It is as if you would open an inner window from which the feeling can now escape ... ... This is how you free yours illness from this feeling ... ... Your body can heal much better now because this feeling is it has now become clear to you ... ... but even if you are not yet sure what feeling it actually is ... ... if you are can't feel it so clearly now ... ... so you know that there is a feeling behind the illness that is now in motion ... ... The feeling is in motion and can now be slowly dissolved ... ... like a warm air stream it can escape through the window inside you ... ... simply dissolve into thin air, because you now know that this feeling exists or gives a feeling that can now be resolved ... ... You no longer need it, because it has long belonged to the Past of ... ... Now the feeling of the illness is released ... ... now disconnected ... ... Now! ... ...

Consolidation (post-hypnotic assignment)

... ... This will make you much more free inside ... ... maybe you can feel it because you can breathe better or you just feel lighter inside ... ... the healing can actually go faster now ... ... really amazing how quickly your body can recover after the deep lying feelings get in motion and be replaced ... ... this is exactly what is happening ... ... detachment ... ... exactly that ... ... detachment ... ... Whenever you concentrate on your body, exactly on that place that should heal again, you give yourself mindfulness and concentrate on this place ... ... So you can strengthen your life force yourself, strengthen your courage, strengthen your hope and also your confidence ... ... so you can experience healing ... ...

Main Part 9: The Flow of Life

Fantasy journey of dreamland therapy (for those affected)

The following hypnosis text works with a fantasy journey (trance story). It means that a sequence of scenes like a little story is chosen as a proxy for that emotional background of the problem dealt with. Dealing with feelings changes attitudes, attitudes and evaluations. Here are the rules of suggestion of less importance than imagination and inner creativity of the client. The pictures are therefore sometimes offered with a lot of details, on the other hand a lot is deliberately left open. This approach is a cooperative type of hypnosis.

...... You have been through a lot lately, taking on the stress of chemotherapy because you decided to go this route of treatment ...... At the same time you go a way of healing, which is also an inner way ...... because deep within you lies the power that you need to get through this time and to recover again and again, between the chemotherapy treatments and after the last session, so that you can then fully recover ... Breathe deeply in and out and relax your muscles ...... your body comes to rest, as if you want to fall asleep to dream a beautiful dream ...... deep in your imagination ...... you pose embark on an inner journey ...... a journey to a faraway country that is also very close ...... The land of your dreams...... Feel the rhythm of your breathing and follow it...... with the wind of your breath you leave your thoughts and go to the land of dreams ...... You are sitting in a meadow that has dried up completely ...... The grass is yellow, almost brown and everything looks very dreary ...... you look around, but everything is so dry here, so drained ...... Then you notice that you are sitting on the bank of a river ...... But the river bed has no water more ...... The power of the river seems to succumb and the meadow that was once there is blooming Life seems interrupted ...... Life seems to stand still ...... You close your eyes and feel your breath ... . you can hear your breath clearly ...... and in the same rhythm your breath also blows the wind gently through the land of dreams ...... you hear the gentle rustling of the wind, which you can soon no longer distinguish from the sound of your breath ...... The sound of your breathing and the wind merge into one another ...... That is breathing and wind same ...... exactly the same ...... And if you focus your attention and all your mindfulness on the sound of the wind, you will hear a soft whisper in the wind ...... a tender voice that speaks to you ...... the wind whispers to you: Everything should bloom ...... Everything should bloom ...... Don't wish it ...... don't long for it come over ...... and then the wind whispers: Just imagine ...... get an idea of it, that's enough ...... And so you follow the words of the wind and imagine how everything will bloom and will find its way back to the old beauty and splendor ...... You imagine how beautiful this one meadow will look like, with lots of flowers and green grass, maybe with friendly animals ... ... with trees that bear sweet fruit ... ... Then you hear the whispering of the wind that tells you: So is it right ... ... That's good ... ... Then you let the picture in your inner eye become clearer ... ... For so long you have only dealt with the fact that the cancer has grown in you ... ... that this disease has spread as if it had been fertilized ... ... But diseases are sometimes there, and we cannot understand why this is happening ... ... We look for explanations and don't find an answer ... ... Then it's time we focused again on what should really grow in us ... ... life should grow ... ... health should grow ... ... hope and joy should grow ... ... because that is exactly what makes our inner world lively and colorful ... ... that is exactly what makes the meadows and fields bloom deep within us ... ... and suddenly you hear rushing water ... ... You open your eyes and look around ... ...water flows through the river bed again ... ... It fills with bubbling water, which afterwards life feels ... ... for progress ... ... for fresh energy ... ... It tears the dry dust of the river bed with itself and turns dark ... ... it's still cloudy, because all the dust and dirt that has accumulated, must first be washed away ... ... But gradually the water becomes clearer and clearer ... ... because life returns ... ... the dust of heavy thoughts and Fears will be washed away ... ... The water gets cleaner and clearer until it finally comes crystal clear and flowing through the river bed ... ... you can see all the way to the bottom ... ... to very deep into the river bed ... ... you can see every stone on the ground ... ... pure, fresh Water ... ... so clear that you can look right down to the bottom of the river bed, very deep down ... ... a beautiful river arises as if by itself ... ... Then you look across the meadow and suddenly small green shoots appear everywhere, emerging from the soil grow so fast that you can watch ... ... grass starts to close before your eyes grow ... ... The meadow suddenly turns green again and everything looks new ... ... It starts to bloom ... ... blooming flowers appear within seconds, nourished by the fresh water of the river in the land of dreams ... ... And so it goes on around you and deep inside you ... ... power blooms ... ... you bloom yourself again ... ... trees suddenly appear on the beautiful meadow, that bear ripe fruit ... ... As in a time lapse, you can watch the watching plants and enjoying them ... ... all of this happens because it is your imagination, because you created a picture of it and put it in front of you looked at your inner eye without expectation ... ... life is back ... ... and also your strength will increase again ... ... You close your eyes and take your body very clearly and consciously true ... ...

Consolidation (post-hypnotic assignment)

... ... You feel that this river of life flows deep inside you and brings new life ...... strength and patience for the upcoming challenges and always new blossoming of your life ... ... You think about the fact that the land of dreams is deep inside you. There was it always. I'm just telling you about it ... ...

Main Part 10: Making Peace

Fantasy journey of dreamland therapy (for those affected who are preparing for the approaching death).

The following hypnosis text works with a fantasy journey (trance story). The explanations in the introductory text on hypnosis 9 apply. This is now about the special task, one to accompany people who only have a short time to live and to offer them an opportunity to make their peace. This can be very special in individual cases. So please take that trance story as a basic idea and lead your client to situations or in special times of his life with which he would like to make his peace. Of course this can trip (or something like that) can be made several times. As a first step, you can become a therapist take the present story, and then tailor others individually to your client. Often three to four sessions have resulted in my peace-making work, until everything what was close to the client's heart had been dealt with. Please do not be afraid to join us soon making imaginary journeys to dying people. People who know and like fantasy journeys are usually open to this form of saying goodbye and even want it actively.

... ... You go to the land of dreams ... ... You stand on a blooming meadow and look into the distance ... ... You can see the entire dreamland; look into a wide valley ... ... And you stand up in the sun ... ... you are here to make your peace ... ... also for yourself to say goodbye, because your time here on earth is coming to an end ... ... You know it, and you are introducing yourself very consciously and actively ... ... here and today, at this very moment ... ... But before you leave this world, you want to make your peace ... ... with unresolved situations ... ... maybe with certain people ... ... you can do today what you still want to clean or lock ... ... maybe that is no longer possible in your waking world, but here in the land of dreams it can happen ... ... dream and reality are only one breath apart ... ... Everything that happens here in the land of dreams happens whole deep in your heart and is reality ... ... your reality, and only that counts ... ... only on it depends ... ... so you go and do this Easter march in the valley of silence ... ... you go down over five large levels into this valley, in which everything is quiet and peaceful ... ... on everyone Level you make peace, if you want it that way ... ... decide for yourself, it is your truth ... ... Your march for peace begins on the fifth level ... ... You look up at the sky and see a message there in bold letters between the clouds. It says: do yours peace now and get free! ... ... Then you come to level four and meet a group of children who play and hardly notice that you are there ... ... One of the children looks the same how you looked when you were a child ... ... it's you yourself, you meet yourself here in one other time, in your childhood ... ... As a visitor to your past, images of earlier times arise around you ... ... a scene is built up that shows you where or with whom in yours childhood you still want to make your peace ... ... Look at the pictures in peace, leave them simply arise and be there, whatever you see, feel or experience ... ... maybe became much has already been cleared up or clarified, and it is possible that much of what happened once remains is, stand like this and can no longer be changed ... ... But you can make your peace now, if you want to ... ... Maybe you want to say something to a person or you just want to be there ... ... do it the way it is right for you, just follow your feeling ... ... take your time until you hear my voice again ... ... *[please give what feels like a minute, then continue]* ... ... Now prepare yourself to continue your Easter march ... ... You go on to the plain three and you arrive in your youth ... ... Here, too, pictures and scenes from that time are created but above all, there are very special events ... ... the events that show you where and with whom you can still make your peace ... ... Take a look at the events and pictures, what however you see or experience ... ... Here too there may be difficult situations, maybe events that have remained open forever ... ... Today you can end them deep in your heart ... ... You can make your peace now, if you want to ... ... Maybe you want to say something to a person or you just want to be there ... ... do it the way it is right for you, just follow your feeling ... ... take your time until you hear my voice again ... ... *[a felt one Please give a minute, then continue]* ... ... Now prepare yourself to continue your Easter march ... ... You go on, deeper and deeper into the valley of silence and come to level two... ... that is the level of your adult life ... ... Here you can find everything again, what you have already lived through as an adult ... ... you can recognize situations, meet people who mean something to you or who have played a major role in your life ... ... some helpful and constructive, others with anger and injustice ... ... Whom or whatever you are meet here, it is right, because you can see where you have not yet made peace ... ... Today you can do it ... ... You can make your peace now, if you want to ... ... Maybe you want to say something to a person or you just want to be there ... ... Do it like this, how it is right for you, just follow your feeling ... ... take your time until you hear my voice like that ... ... *[please give what feels like a minute, then continue]* ... ... prepare yourself now before to continue your Easter march ... ... You go further into the deep valley and come to one on the level ... ... Here you meet the person who is most important to you in life ... ... Possibly there is nothing unexplained with this person ... ... maybe everything has been discussed and everything is understood between you ... ... but maybe there is still something uncleaned here and there ... ... You can either make your peace with everything that is still open with this dear person is or with everything that could possibly be open without your knowing it ... ... But even if everything is already in order ... ... you can make your peace together ... ... make peace with her illness ... ... peace with fate ... ... peace with God, if you can believe in him, or just peace with another authority in which you can believe ... ... you can now yours make peace, if you want it that way ... ... Maybe you want to say something to a person or you want to say something to God ... ... do it the way it is right for you, just follow your feeling ... ... take your time until you hear my voice again ... ... *[please give what feels like a minute, then continue]* ... ... Now prepare to continue your Easter march ... ... Finally you go all the way through the valley of silence and meet yourself at the end of the valley ... ... you meet yourself like a twin sister / brother and make peace with yourself now ... ... You forgive yourself for everything you have ever accused yourself of ... ... You treat yourself with respect and dignity and thank yourself for everything you have tried in your life, for all that you have succeeded in and also for what you have not succeeded, because you have yours Humanity shown ... ... Make your peace with yourself now ... ... Do it as it is for you is correct, just follow your feeling ... ... take your time until you hear my voice again ... ... *[Please give what feels like a minute, then continue]* ... ...

Transition to rejection 1:

… … Now you will soon wake up, and your organism is preparing for it … … Take your time and slowly prepare to come back to life … … at your own pace … … to fill your body with life at your own pace … … your mind and yours to fill the spirit with life … … to become and remain fully alive and awake again … … to come and stay fully alive and awake … … *[If body signals were used, the suggestions in question should be withdrawn. "You have full control over your arm and your fingers".]* … … You feel the connection to your body and you are aware that body and spirit now start the way back into waking life … …

Transition to rejection 2:

… … Soon you have to wake up completely … … return to your everyday life and act actively … … We have reached the end of your inner journey today … … a journey that led you to yourself to find strength and courage … … to recognize that you have a lot can hold out what you might not have believed you could do … … But now you're back full of trust and strength … … So now you come back to the present of the moment … … The journey is over and maybe this very end is also the beginning of something completely new and beautiful … … Now it is important that you are fully awake again … … Now it is time to get back to the moment of the present and get into the orienting space into it by both of us being …

… … *[If body signals were used, the suggestions in question should be withdrawn. "You have full control over your arm and your fingers".]* … …

My voice guides you, shows you the way back … … You hear me clearly and clearly and just follow my voice that brings you back … …

Transition to diversion 3:

... ... Now just let go of all inner images slowly ... ... All images dissolve like a fog, which slowly disappears and brings you a clear and new look ... ... Let your thoughts just go back and forth ... ... let it wander and let go of all the pictures ... ... stand up to wake up soon and then to be free and open to new thoughts ... ... free and open ... ... enough has been done for today ... ... enough is done for today ... ... you now stand on it to be woken up again soon ... ...

> ... ... *[If body signals were used, the suggestions in question should be withdrawn. "You have full control over your arm and your fingers".]* ... ...

Move your arms and legs very consciously and inform your body that it should now adjust to activity and movement, alertness and clarity ... ... good so ......

Rejection 1:

... ... The time has come. You have to wake up now. I count to seven and when I get to seven, and then you are completely awake. Completely awake and well rested. As soon as I get to seven you are completely awake and just open your eyes ... ...

- ... One ... your body wakes up ...
- ... Two ... you start moving ...
- ... Three ... your hearing becomes sharper. You hear me clearly ...
- ... Four ... Your body feels normal and good, you have full control over your body ...
- ... Five ... you become more awake and awake ...
- ... Six ... my voice is getting louder ...
- ... Seven ... you are awake! Open eyes! ... ...

Rejection 2:

... ... Your body is filled with life and strength. You will become more alert from your feet to your head. The waking up starts with your feet. Your feet wake up and move. Maybe you feel it is a little clearer again. Then your legs wake up and move, first your lower thighs and then your thighs. You move your legs. Then your stomach can wake up and your back wakes up too. Your upper body moves as a sign of waking up. You feel the pad under your body. Your upper body becomes more alert and alert. Also yours arms wake up and move. You can now stretch and stretch yourself. Finally yours wakes up head up. Your thoughts become clearer and you want to open your eyes. You come back and are awake. You open your eyes now! ... ...

Rejection 3:

... ... I am bringing you back to waking life now. Focus on your hearing. Then you will feel that the noises of the surroundings become clearer. You can orient yourself with your ears and pick up exactly all the noises that are here in this room. It's like testing your hearing louder and waking up in the process. So turn up the volume, then listen you make me louder ... ... *[They get louder when speaking so that the client can understand the effect.]* ......Next, focus on your sense of touch. You can see your surroundings above your body feel. Then you feel, for example, the pad under your body. You can also use the grab it with your hands and feel the pad. This sense also works great and you wake up. Then focus on your eyes. You can already with closed eyes recognize some light shining through your eyelids. To make this sense even more intensify, you now slowly open your eyes. Open your eyes. You know your surroundings see again and be awake ... ...

Book series coming soon

Volume 1: Psychooncology
Volume 2: Psychosomatic Disorders
Volume 3: Burn Out
Volume 4: Tinnitus
Volume 5: chronic pain
Volume 6: Migraines and Chronic Headaches
Volume 7: Obesity, Eating Addiction
Volume 8: restless legs
Volume 9: Anxiety and Restlessness
Volume 10: Thoughts of Suicide and Attempted Suicide
Volume 11: Depressive Thoughts
Volume 12: panic attacks
Volume 13: drug abuse
Volume 14: Blockage solution and positive thinking
Volume 15: Stress Reduction, Stress Management
Volume 16: workaholic
Volume 17 nervous breakdown
Volume 18: Coming to terms with the past
Volume 19: Mourning Work
Volume 20: Addictive Tendencies

www.ingramcontent.com/pod-product-compliance
Lightning Source LLC
Chambersburg PA
CBHW070312220526
45465CB00004B/1854